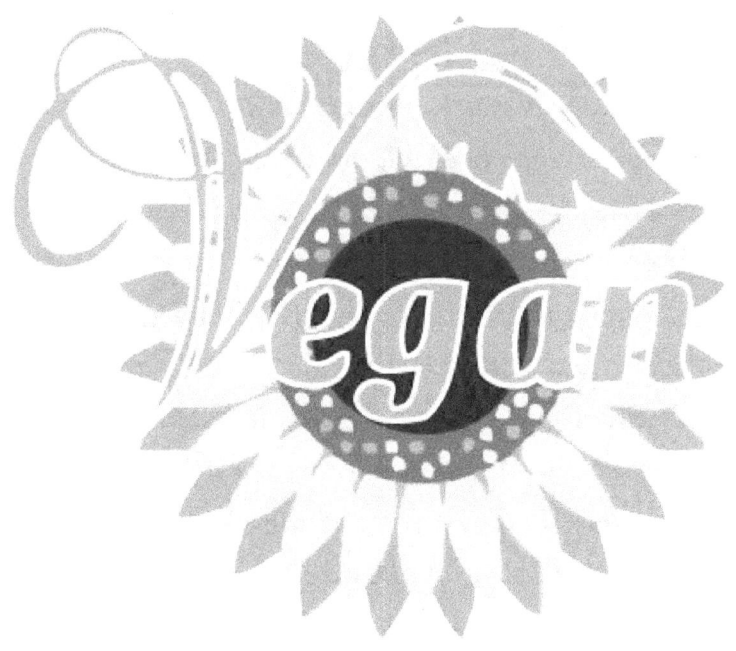

Introduction

Being a vegan is much more than a dietary choice simply just to eat healthily and enjoy your food; it is a movement towards compassion and love for the beings on earth. It is recognition for the pain, abuse and suffering that many animals around the world face every day and a decision not to play any part in the continuation of this suffering. It is truly a beautiful gesture for any human being to make and one that has the power to radically change the way people feel, in terms of their health and wellbeing, and also transform a person's perception of the world which leads to a deeper connection to all life.

When a person becomes vegan a whole new and exciting world opens up and suddenly they feel a part of a much wider movement of sensitive and caring people. On a very deep level there will always be a deep respect and understanding of other vegans in a way that makes people feel as though they are part of one big family. Across the world there are approximately 170million vegans and the number is growing every day as veganism as a way of life is quickly on the increase. Many people are waking up to the plight of the animals on this earth today and are choosing love and compassion over violence and greed.

So, welcome to the world of veganism, and well done on making a choice that is compassionate, loving, kind and considerate. Your choice is helping the world in so many ways, which will later be explained. Peace and love to you sweet vegan friend, peace and love. Namaste.

Contents

Omnivores, Carnivores or Herbivores?

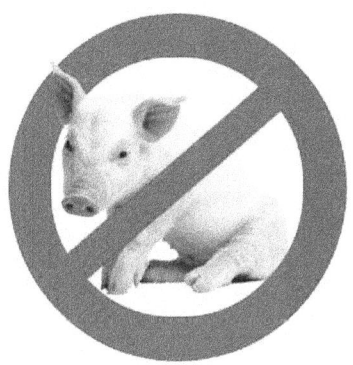

A question often asked by many; often part of the confusion in our society today is caused by this notion that humans are designed to animals, and eating animals has become a huge social and cultural norm that is widely accepted by many as being 'natural'. Well, there is lots and lots of scientific proof that suggests otherwise, and here is some of it;

Carnivores: have claws

Herbivores: no claws

Humans: no claws

Carnivores: have no skin pores and perspire through the tongue

Herbivores: perspire through skin pores

Humans: perspire through skin pores

Carnivores: have sharp front teeth for tearing, with no flat molar teeth for grinding

Herbivores: no sharp front teeth, but flat rear molars for grinding

Humans: no sharp front teeth, but flat rear molars for grinding

Carnivores: have intestinal tract that is only 3 times their body length so that rapidly decaying meat can pass through quickly

Herbivores: have intestinal tract 10-12 times their body length.

Humans: have intestinal tract 10-12 times their body length.

Carnivores: have strong hydrochloric acid in stomach to digest meat

Herbivores: have stomach acid that is 20 times weaker than that of a meat-eater

Humans: have stomach acid that is 20 times weaker than that of a meat-eater

Carnivores: salivary glands in mouth not needed to pre-digest grains and fruits.

Herbivores: well-developed salivary glands which are necessary to pre-digest grains and fruits

Humans: well-developed salivary glands, which are necessary to pre-digest, grains and fruits

Carnivores: have acid saliva with no enzyme ptyalin to pre-digest grains

Herbivores: have alkaline saliva with ptyalin to pre-digest grains

Humans: have alkaline saliva with ptyalin to pre-digest grains

Health and wellbeing

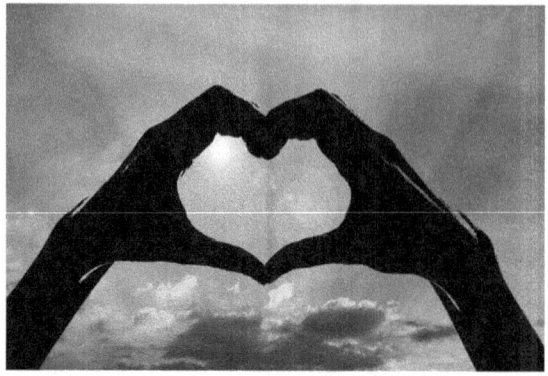

Health defects from consumption of animals and health benefits from being vegan;

Eating animal products and health

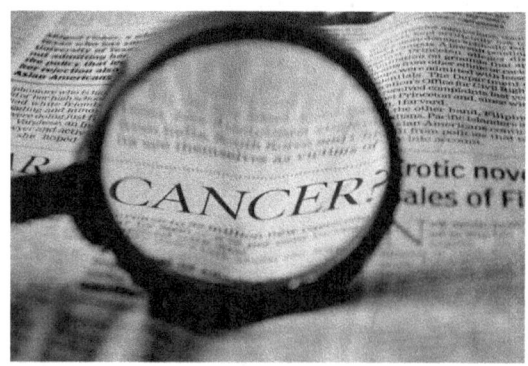

There is the view in the world that eating animals and animal products is actually good for your health—here is just some of the evidence to suggest otherwise; (see references for source studies)

Inflammation. Arachidonic acid (found in animal foods) is linked to brain inflammation, depression, anxiety, and stress. Arachidonic acid is used by our bodies to create inflammation. Our bodies produce all the arachidonic acid we need unlike other animals (e.g. cats) who produce little to none because their bodies expect to get theirs from their diet (meat). Excess arachidonic acid means excess inflammation. Chicken and eggs are the top sources of arachidonic acid. A single meal of high-fat animal products has been shown to spike inflammation within hours that can stiffen one's arteries.

Bacterial toxins. Significant levels of bacterial toxins are found in animal products that cause endotoxemia (bacterial toxins in the bloodstream) within hours of eating. Bacteria endotoxins from animal products have been shown to survive high heat cooking for long periods, acid (like our stomachs), and digestive enzymes.

Eggs, cancer and bodily dysfunction. Only Half an egg a day or more is shown to double the odds of mouth, throat, esophageal, prostate, and bladder cancer; triple the odds of colon and breast cancer. Also, 14%

of retail eggs contain viruses of the leukosis/sarcoma group. One egg contains almost 2/3 of the cholesterol limit suggested by the American Heart Association for healthy people.

Many types of cancer. Nitrites in processed meat form nitrosamines (carcinogens also found in cigarette smoke) and are associated with the two leading pediatric cancers, brain tumors and childhood leukemia. Processed meat is greatly associated with stomach, colon, rectum, pancreatic, lung, prostate, testicular, kidney, and bladder cancer. Dietary fat of animal origin is linked to pancreatic cancer, And all types of meat (no matter how it is cooked) increases the risk of cancer of the uterus. And Cured meat seems to increase the chance of getting chronic obstructive pulmonary disease (COPD)

Contamination. 47% of U.S. retail meat tested is contaminated with Staphylococcus bacteria. Multidrug resistant strains were common.

Allergies. Animal consumption increases allergies including asthma, bee stings, drug allergies, and hayfever.

Blood cancer. Poultry consumption is associated with an increase in lymphoma (blood cancer) and prostate enlargement.

Bowel problems. Animal flesh, fish, cheese, and general animal protein intake have been associated with an increased risk of inflammatory bowel disease (IBD). And dairy intake can double your risk of heart attack.

Kidney dysfunction. Kidney failure is linked to animal flesh consumption and has been shown to cause human proteins to be urinated out (microalbuminuria). Something that should never happen naturally. Animal flesh is acidic which causes higher risk of kidney stones and lower urine acid clearance.

Metabolic dysfunction. Meat eaters have a lower resting metabolism compared to vegans also, Even when looking at endurance athletes, meat eaters' arteries are thicker (from atherosclerosis plaque) than your average vegan.

So basically eating meat has been linked to many types of health problems including cancer, disease, organ malfunction and metabolic abnormality, which makes you wonder, if eating animal products was

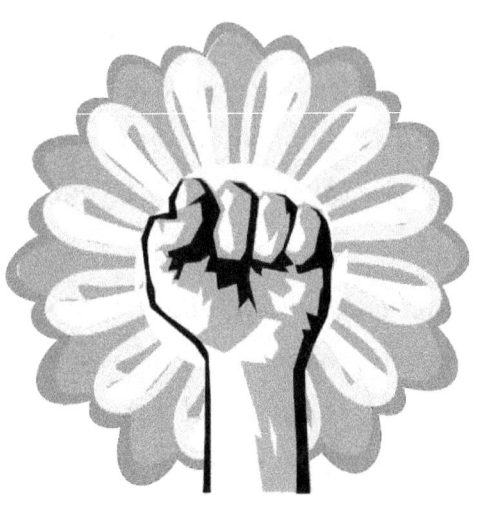

Fibre. A diet high in fibre (especially found in fruits and vegetables) leads to healthier bowel movements. High fibre diets help fight against colon cancer.

Magnesium. Aiding in the absorption of calcium, magnesium is an often overlooked vitamin in importance to a healthy diet. Nuts, seeds, and dark leafy greens are an excellent source of magnesium.

Potassium. Potassium balances water and acidity in your body and stimulates the kidneys to eliminate toxins. Diets high in potassium have shown to reduce the risk of cardiovascular diseases and cancer.

Folate. This B vitamin is an important part of a healthy diet. Folate helps with cell repair, generating red and white blood cells, and metabolizing amino acids.

Antioxidants. For protection against cell damage, antioxidants are one of the best ways to help your body. Many researchers also believe that antioxidants help protect your body against forming many types of cancer.

Vitamin C. Boosts your immune system and helps keep your gums healthy and heal faster. Vitamin C is also an antioxidant.

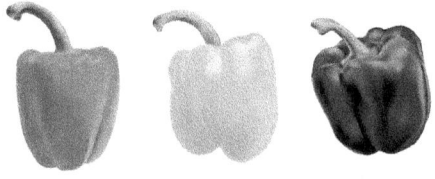

strokes, as you're not filling yourself with saturated fats and cholesterol.

Cholesterol. Remove any food that comes from an animal and you will remove all dietary cholesterol from your diet!

Blood pressure. A diet rich in whole grains is beneficial to your health in many ways. A major advantage is lowering high blood pressure.

Type 2 diabetes. A vegan diet significantly reduces the chance of developing diabetes.

Prostate cancer. It has been shown that men in the early stages of prostate cancer who switched to a vegan diet either stopped the progress of the cancer or may have even reversed the illness.

Colon cancer. Eating a diet consisting of whole grains, along with fresh fruits and vegetables, can greatly reduce your chances of colon cancer.

Breast cancer. Countries where women eat very little animal products have a much lower rate of breast cancer than do the women in countries that consume more animal products.

Macular degeneration. Diets with lots of fresh fruits and vegetables, especially leafy greens, carrots, pumpkin, and sweet potatoes, can help prevent the onset of age-related macular degeneration. (Age related macular degeneration is a medical condition that results in a loss of vision in the centre of the visual field because of damage to the retina.)

Cataracts. cataracts are also prevented through the intake of fruits and vegetables. Produce high in antioxidants also help prevent cataracts.

Arthritis. Eliminating dairy consumption will alleviate arthritis symptoms.

Osteoporosis. Bone health depends on a balance of protein, adequate calcium intake, high potassium, and low sodium, with a healthy vegan diet this is achieved. High protein intake will leach the bones of calcium in attempts to digest the dense amino acids. This is especially important for women over 50.

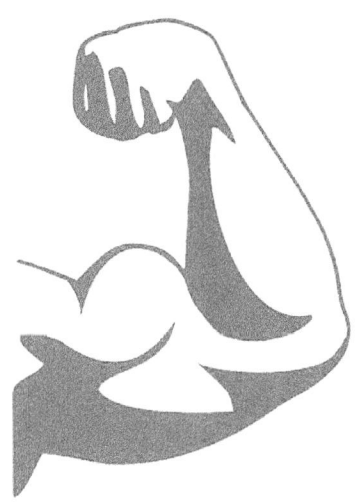

Longer life. Those following the vegan way of life live an average of 10 to 15 years longer than those who do not.

Body odor. Removing dairy and animal flesh from the diet significantly reduces body odor. Going vegan means smelling better.

Bad breath. It has been found that vegans have fewer breath and mouth issues.

Hair. Hair becomes stronger, has more body, and looks healthier.

Nails. Healthy vegan diets also create much stronger, healthier nails. Due in part to the heart healthy fats in nuts such as Omega-2. Nail health is said to be an indicator of overall health.

PMS. many women tell how PMS symptoms become much less intense or disappear altogether. The elimination of dairy is thought to help with those suffering with PMS as diary contains hormones, which creates an imbalance in the human body.

Migraines. Migraine suffers who go on vegan diets often discover relief from their migraines.

Allergies. Reduction in dairy, animal flesh and eggs is often tied to alleviation of allergies.

So from the evidence it is clear that it is widely accepted and known that a healthy vegan diet provides you with optimum health and wellbeing and will give you everything your body needs, even vitamin B12 which can be found in soy products, and yeast extracts! So why then do animals have to suffer and die? Answer; habit, tradition, greed, profiteering, capitalism, indulgence. It is not necessary to hurt and kill animals for health and survival; it is a choice that is made and a choice that can be changed. When people choose vegan it will affect the needs of the consumer and in turn affect what businesses sell. If people choose vegan, businesses will supply vegan, unless they want to go bankrupt.

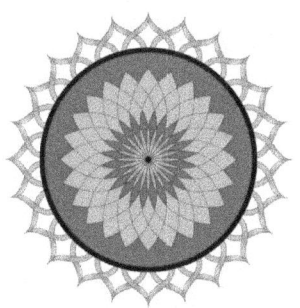

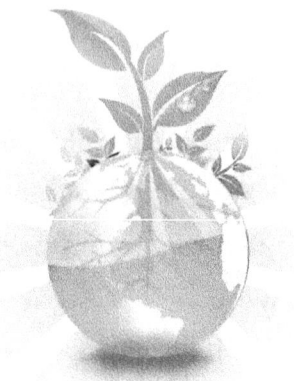

It takes 2,500 gallons of water to produce a pound of meat but only 25 gallons to produce a pound of wheat.

Producing just one hamburger uses enough fossil fuel to drive a small car 20 miles! Of all raw materials and fossil fuels used in the U.S., more than one-third are devoted to raising animals for food.

A typical pig factory generates the same amount of raw waste as a city of 12,000 people. According to the Environmental Protection Agency, raising animals for food is the number-one source of water pollution.

Of all agricultural land in the U.S., 87% is used to raise animals for food. That's 45% of the total land mass in the U.S. About 260 million acres of U.S. forest have been cleared to create cropland to produce feed for animals raised for food. The animal flesh industry is directly responsible for 85% of all soil erosion in the U.S.

More than 80% of the corn we grow and more than 95% of the oats are fed to livestock. The world's cattle alone consume a quantity of food equal to the caloric needs of 8.7 billion people—more than the entire human population on Earth. According to the Worldwatch Institute Roughly 2 of every 5 tons of grain produced in the world is fed to livestock, poultry, or fish; decreasing consumption of these products, especially from cows, could free up massive quantities of grain to feed the starving, end food shortages and reduce massive pressures on the land.

A German study conducted in 2008 concluded that a meat-eater's diet is responsible for more than seven times as much greenhouse-gas emissions as a vegan's diet is, showing that if you care about the planet and your carbon footprint veganism is the only option.

So, it's clear, that choosing to go vegan will not only benefit you, but it will also benefit the planet. And in benefiting the planet you will benefit every living thing on earth. And choosing to go vegan not only benefits everything on the planet it also helps to stop large scale abuse, pain, torture and suffering to the billions of animals that are enslaved to produce food each year. Did you know that on average, just by going vegan you will save the lives of around 200 animals every year, times that by approximately 170million and you can see just what a wonderful and inspiring impact veganism is having on the planet.

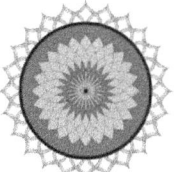

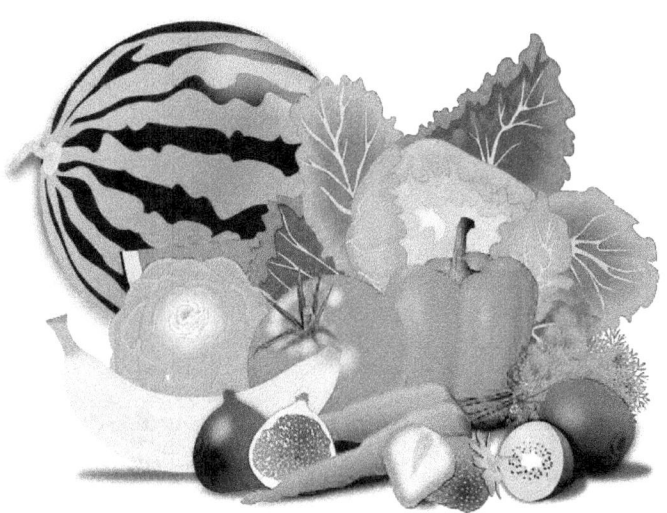

Calcium

broccoli, green leafy vegetables (such as kale, bok choy, collard and turnip greens), tofu, blackstrap molasses, chickpeas, many beans, sesame seeds, sunflower seeds, almonds, flax seeds, brazil nuts, dried figs, dried fruit.

Iron

green leafy vegetables & sea vegetables, legumes/beans, nuts & seeds, blackstrap molasses, dried fruits, watermelon, prune juice, spinach, cereals, whole grains.

Magnesium

brown rice, cooked spinach, beans/legumes, almonds/nuts, dried figs, broccoli, cooked oatmeal, wheat germ/bran, whole grains, green leafy vegetables, bananas, peanuts.

Phosphorus

pinto beans, cereal grains, almonds, nuts, dried beans, peas, lentils, peanuts, brown rice, avocados, spinach, many vegetables, yeast.

Potassium

raisins, bananas, raw and cooked spinach, potatoes, baked sweet potatoes, winter squash, raw cauliflower, avocados, kiwifruit, dried fruits, tomatoes, oranges, grapefruit, strawberries, honeydew melon, cantaloupe, dried apricots.

Zinc

pumpkin seeds, whole grains/cereals, legumes, lentils, peas, soy foods, nuts, sunflower seeds, wheat germ, yeast, garbanzo beans, raw collard greens, spinach, corn.

Selenium

brazil nuts, whole grains, kidney beans (depending on the soil they are grown in), yeast.

Manganese

brown rice & whole grains, cereals, cooked oatmeal, wheat germ, nuts, seeds, legumes, cooked spinach & kale, black beans, almonds, avocados, pineapples, strawberries.

Molybdenum

beans, breads, cereals, cooked spinach, strawberries.

Pantothenic Acid

whole grain cereals, legumes, mushrooms, peanuts, soybeans, avocados, sunflower seeds, bananas, oranges, cooked collard greens, baked potato, broccoli.

Chromium

whole grains, nuts, broccoli, apples, peanuts, cooked spinach, mushrooms.

Biotin

cereals & whole grains, breads, yeast, almonds, peanuts, molasses, legumes.

Copper

nuts and seeds, whole grains, dried beans, mushrooms.

Folic Acid

legumes, lentils, oranges, whole grains, asparagus, spinach, romaine lettuce.

Iodine

iodine-rich sea vegetables, kelp, vegetables grown in iodine-rich soil.

Protein

Beans, lentils, nuts, seeds, many vegetables including broccoli, tofu, soy.

Vitamin A

carrots, winter squashes (acorn and butternut), sweet potatoes, cantaloupe, apricots, spinach, kale, turnip greens, broccoli, red bell peppers and other greens.

Vitamin B1 (Thiamin)

brown rice & whole grains, bread, pasta, oatmeal, brewers and nutritional yeast, legumes, cereals, sunflower seeds, nuts, watermelon, raw wheat germ.

Riboflavin

yeast, beans, cereals, whole grains, spinach, broccoli, wheat germ, mushrooms.

Vitamin B3 (Niacin)

legumes, brown rice, green vegetables, potatoes, tomatoes, broccoli.

Vitamin B6

whole grains, peanuts, nuts/legumes, soybeans, walnuts, bananas, watermelon

Vitamin C

bell peppers, broccoli, tomatoes, strawberries, oranges/orange juice, grapefruit, tomatoes, brussel sprouts, cabbage, collard greens, turnip greens, spinach, potatoes, melon, berries, papayas, romaine lettuce, watercress.

Vitamin D

The most significant supply of Vitamin D comes from sunlight exposure on the skin. Vitamin D-2 supplements are available, as well as Vitamin D fortified plant milks & cereals. Fortified vegan products contain Vitamin D-2 (ergocalciferol) as opposed to animal-derived Vitamin D-3 (cholecalciferol).

Vitamin E

vegetable oils, sunflower seeds, raw wheat germ, nuts, peanuts, green leafy vegetables, whole wheat flour, whole grains, spinach.

Vitamin K

green leafy vegetables, spinach, turnip greens, kale, parsley, brussel sprouts, broccoli, cauliflower, soybeans and soybean oil, cabbage, green tea, tomatoes.

Vitamin B12

Nutritional Yeast, B-12 fortified non-dairy milks and cereals. Vegan B-12 supplements, fermented soy products and supplements.

<u>Veganism and Spirituality</u>

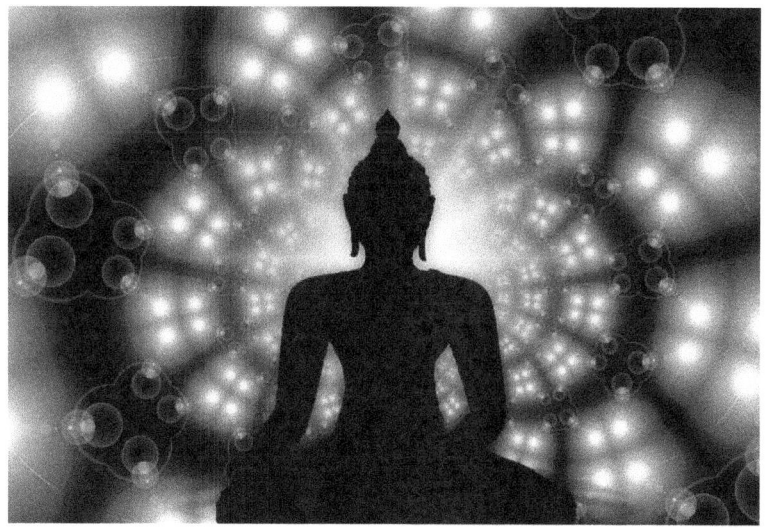

Being a vegan is far more than just a diet, it is a commitment to peace and spiritual wellbeing. Being vegan is beneficial for the earth, for nature and for everything that lives and will help you along your spiritual path. So because being a vegan is in its

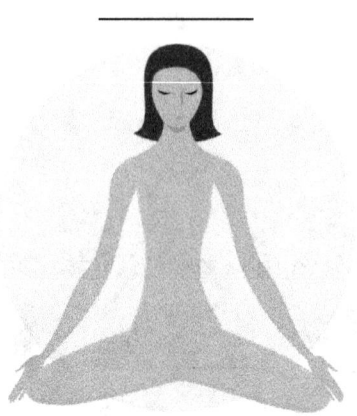

There are many ways in which you can practice meditation, and to begin with it is a good idea to practice getting used to and comfortable with doing 'nothing', just being still and just simply observing, observing your senses, your breath, your emotions, the world around you, sights, sounds and smells and just being with it, just observing.

Do this regularly for 10-15 minutes each day and see how you feel.

Next, you might like to close your eyes and sit still and just continue to observe, just in a state of 'non-doing' just simply 'being'. If you find that your mind is racing and you have lots of thoughts, that's ok, just observe, and allow the thoughts, everything is normal, and you will always be 'doing it right' as there is no 'wrong way'.

Next, you might like to try getting a little more focused, and just bringing all of your attention on to your breath, just breathing and feeling, putting all of your focus on how it feels to breathe. You could even count your breaths to keep the mind focused, counting repeatedly from zero to ten. Or you might wish to just count the out-breath, or just the in-breath. The important thing is to just stay focused on breathing and how it feels. How does it feel for the air to be passing into your mouth and nose, follow the air down into your lungs, down into the bottom of your stomach, also, try to breathe with your belly not with your chest i.e. physically and consciously move your lower belly to draw in the air instead of using your chest, with enough practice this will become habit. Breathing in this way actually reduces stress by the effect it has on your nervous system.

Stick with the breath meditation for a while until you really feel the benefit. Eventually breathing will become something that will fill your body with peace every time you breathe and it will feel more and more pleasurable over time.

Next you might like to go a little deeper and meditate on the question 'who am I'. In our lives we often build up an elaborate picture of ourselves and what we think we are, when actually we might not be those things, this question will further help you with your meditation and will help to tune you in more and more to the profound alive silent self that is inside you and is deeply entwined and interwoven into the fabric of the universe and everything in it. Eventually when you as yourself this question 'who am I' in your meditations, you might reach a point where the mind doesn't respond, there is just silence, and also you feel ok about that, like you don't need an answer any more. That silence is enough, and that silence is satisfying. This is a very good stage to get to with your meditations.

Next you might wish to incorporate your meditations into daily life and how you interact with the world and with others. This practice of just allowing life to unfold, and allowing yourself to think anything you like, feel whatever you like, behave in any way you like, trusting yourself to be yourself, is a good stage of spiritual growth. Just observe yourself, be aware, and be centred inside yourself.

Finding peace inside of oneself is a wonderful thing for any vegan to do, your diet will naturally create a lot of peace and harmony inside you and your energy will be healthy and strong, but meditation will also be beneficial and will further help you to create and spread peace and love into the world and throughout your own body and mind.

Guided Meditations

Guided meditations can be a great thing to practice with other people. If there is two of you, one person would meditate, while the other reads the guided meditation. If there is a group of you, just have one person read whilst everyone else meditates.

Here is a guided meditation to try with your friends. Read it slowly. You can add your own touches too if you wish.

Meditation

Find a place where you can be still for a while, either sitting or lying down. Close your eyes and just let go. Let go of everything, and just be here, now, in this room, listening to my voice. Watch your thoughts and your feelings and just allow. Allow anything to drift through, like clouds in the sky, your thoughts are just passing through, just watch them. Become aware of your breath, and notice how it feels to breathe. Air passing into your nose and mouth and down, deep down into your belly, and then up and back out through the nose and back into the room. Just observe and feel the breath cycle and allow the breath to fill your body with peace, relaxation and gentleness.

Just breathe. Slowly. Gently. Breathing. Observing. Feeling.

Breathing.

Now imagine that you are stood in a garden. The grass is bright green and the air is filled with the beautiful fragrance of summer flowers. There are trees in the garden and lots of brightly coloured, pretty flowers. You begin to walk, and as you walk you begin to hear the sound of a harp playing in the distance. The notes soft and gentle, the music is beautiful. You walk towards the sound and see a beautiful angelic being playing the harp; you walk over to the being and sit down. You listen to the music for a while and just observe. You look at the sky, the trees and the flowers and feel the wind gently blowing around you. The music is sweet and very healing, it soothes you deeply and you feel as though the music is flowing into you, nourishing you, filling your body with peaceful vibrations.

The music then comes to an end and there is a peaceful, yet vibrantly alive silence. The air is still and the leaves on the trees are still. The being looks towards you and holds out its hand. There is a gift for you in the angel's hand. You take the gift and place it in your pocket. You hug the angel and feel the warmth of the angels love surround you. You stand up and walk away slowly, the angel smiles and waves and then begins to play the harp again.

You walk into the distance and enter a large field with lots of open and empty space. You walk into the centre of the field and sit down. You feel the love of your heart inside of you and you close your eyes and feel it deeply. This love begins to grow stronger and stronger, you feel it growing and it begins to flow through your body and out into your aura. The love is limitless and flows endlessly like an endless river, flowing and flowing. This love filters into the earth surrounding you, into the flowers and the plants, into the insects and into the sky. The love grows and grows, into the atmosphere, until it reaches all beings, your love envelopes all beings, all life, your peace is spreading and flowing into all life and into the whole planet. You feel love deeply, inside and out, your love is flowing, into space, into the universe, forever in time. Love. Peaceful, gentle, light. Love. Life-force. All beings. All life. Peace. Love.

You stand and you walk, back towards the trees. Into the garden full of flowers. You smell the sweet fragrance. You feel the wind around you.

Now, slowly, gently, bring your attention back to your breath. Breathing softly into your belly. Filling your body with beautiful divine breath. Filling you with life-force, vitality, peace. Bring your attention back to your breath, and now to your body. Feel your feet, your legs. Your stomach, your chest. Your hands, your arms. Your shoulders, your neck. And now feel your face and the top of your head. And when you are ready, in your own time, slowly, gently come back into the room. Wiggle your hands and your feet and have a good stretch if you need to.

<u>The end.</u>

Now, you might wish to talk about your experiences and ask each other about the appearance of the angelic being, and also what the gift was. It will be different for everyone.

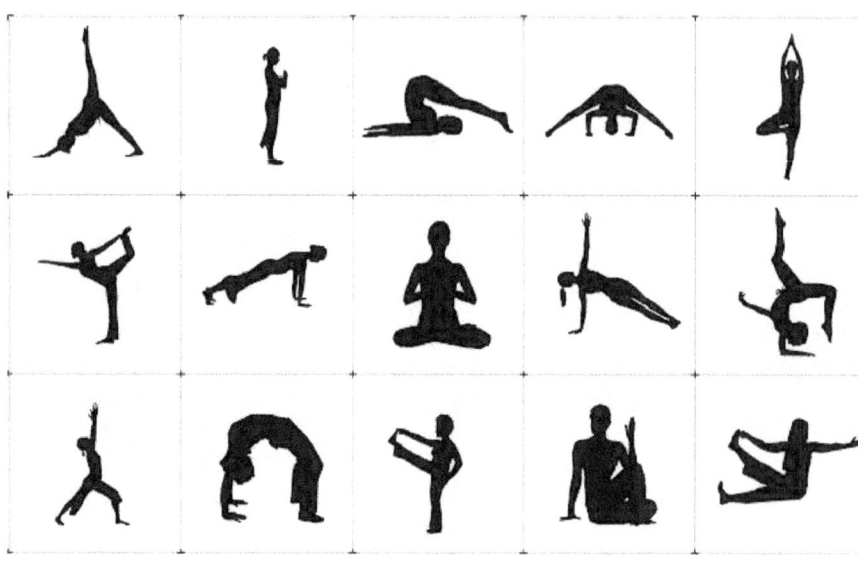

Yoga and the energetic body

Within many esoteric traditions there is thought to be a number of different energetic systems within the body that control the flow of Prana (life force) throughout the body. These systems are also thought to bridge the gap between the physical world and the spiritual world, and link us to the eternal and divine. Perhaps the most well known system is the Chakra system.

Chakras are points within the body where there is a high concentration of energy. There is commonly thought to be seven main points within the body that run up through the centre, starting from the coccyx (tail bone) and working right up into the crown of the head. The first chakra found at the root of the body near the tail bone is known as the 'Meuladhara' and is thought of as a 4 petal lotus flower, red in colour and is the centre of primal grounded instincts. Next is the 'Svadhistana' (the abode of the self) found in the sacrum, is thought of as a 6 petal lotus and is orange in colour and is linked to creativity. Next is the 'Manipura' (the abode of gems) found in the solar plexus, considered to be a 10 petal lotus and yellow in colour – thought to be the centre of willpower. Next the 'Anahata' (unsounded sound) found in the heart, seen as a 12 petal lotus, green in colour and is the centre of compassion. Next is the 'vishudi' (purification) found in the throat, is seen as a 16 petal lotus and is purple/blue in colour, centre for communication. Next the 'Ajna' (control) a two petal lotus found in the third eye, is considered to be silver in colour and is the centre for intuition. And finally the 'Sahasara' (thousand) found on the crown of the head, thought of as a thousand petal lotus and is the centre for union with the divine, the infinite.

Another energetic system that plays a role within Yoga is the meridian system of energy flow. Found throughout the body, the meridian lines travel to every part of the body and it is thought that these lines can get blocked. Yoga postures can help stretch the body and release blockages found within the meridian lines helping the flow of Prana circulate well. It is often worth considering when planning a Yoga class if you wish to target certain areas of the body which postures to practice to open up and unblock certain meridian lines.

As part of your spiritual practice when being a vegan, it can be good to incorporate some yoga postures into your overall programme for mental and physical wellbeing.

Here is a sequence called the 'Sun Salutation' and it is a great one to practice;

Getting Active

Once a person has woken up to the pain, suffering and exploitation of animals by humans and made the conscious movement towards compassion by becoming vegan, it is important to try and inform others or to somehow contribute towards the end of animal exploitation. This can be done in many ways, and once you start to travel down this path you will see that veganism is a large social movement with many people who feel just the same as you do.

Getting involved with animal welfare groups such as PETA, Mercy for animals or action aid is a great way to be part of the solution. You could become a leaflet distributer and encourage the spreading of information and truth. You could also visit schools and colleges and place up information about veganism and animal exploitation on notice boards. You could also offer to give talks similar to the very inspiring animal rights activist Gary Yourofsky.

If you are creative, maybe you could also paint pictures, or make songs about veganism and animal rights and post them on social networks on the internet. You could start a blog and also create pages on many of the internet's social networks.

You could start a vegan 'meet-up' group and get together with other vegans. Maybe you could organise a peaceful protest, showing how you feel about the exploitation of animals in any way that you can think of. Getting the attention of the people and helping people to realise fully the truth of what is happening to billions of animals all around the world every year, is a truly worthy and noble cause, and one which will open up the minds, hearts and eyes of people to see the truth of what's really happening.

Maybe you could organise a screening of many of the recent animal rights and information films that have recently been released, such as 'Earthlings' or 'Cowspiricy'. You could also show some of the many films that PETA make. There is also a whole range of vegan clothing that you could wear with pro-vegan messages on the front, this is a subtle and effective way of just spreading the message as you go about your day. By getting active, you will be saving lives and making a huge difference, and from one vegan to another, I thank you for caring, and for doing something to help the animals.

Tasty Vegan recipes

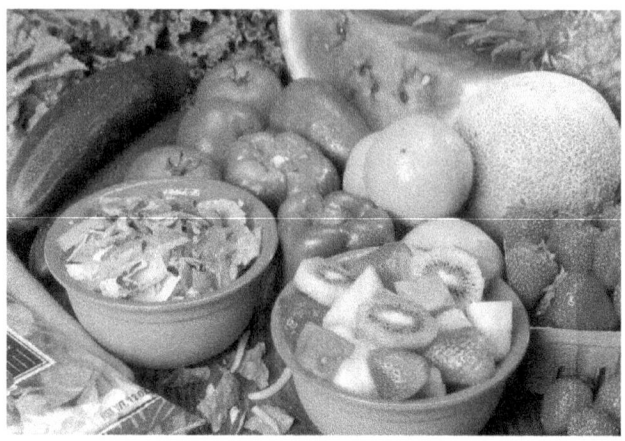

Vegetable curry

Ingredients:

440g/1lb sweet potatoes, chopped

2 tbsp sunflower oil

1 onion, chopped

1 red pepper, chopped

440g/1lb peas

225g/8oz green beans

1 tsp cumin seeds

1 tsp fennel seeds

1 tsp mustard seeds

1 tsp turmeric powder

2 cloves of garlic

½-1 tsp chilli powder, according to taste

1 can coconut milk

1 can of chopped tomatoes

1 can of chickpeas

2 tsp tomato puree

1 tsp veg stock (add to taste)

Method:

1. add all veg to pan and fry with seeds and spices.

2. add can of coconut milk and tomatoes and tomato puree and chickpeas

3. add veg stock and chilli and cook until veg is soft.

4. serve with boiled rice and garnish with fresh coriander and maybe side salad.

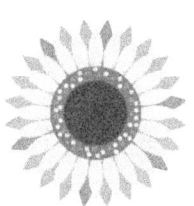

Vegetable risotto with creamy mushroom sauce

Ingredients:

2 cups of risotto rice

1 red pepper

2 white onion

1 courgette

10 cherry tomatoes

440g peas

Veg stock

Italian herbs

White wine

Soy cream

4 cloves of garlic

10 chestnut mushrooms

10 sticks of asparagus

Method:

1. chop all veg except one onion and 2 cloves of garlic.

2. add chopped veg to pan and fry lightly.

3. add 700ml of boiling water to the pan with the frying veg.

4. add risotto rice and veg stock to water and veg.

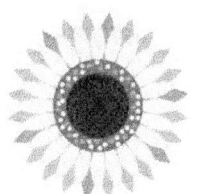

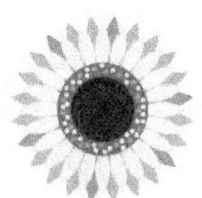

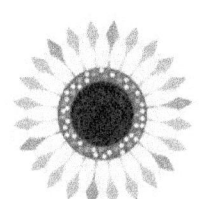

1 tbsp turmeric

½ tsp mild chilli powder

2 cup red lentils

3 cups water (add more during cooking time if you prefer more runny dahl)

1 tin chopped tomatoes

Juice ½ lemon

Veg stock to taste

Method:

1. Wash lentils well in a sieve before adding them to a pan with water.

2. Bring to boil before simmering, while you prepare the spice mix (step 3).

3. while the lentils cook, In a separate pan, fry onion, garlic for a minute in the sunflower oil, before adding the cumin, fennel, mustard seeds, turmeric and chilli. Brown off for a minute or two, stirring, but don't allow to burn.

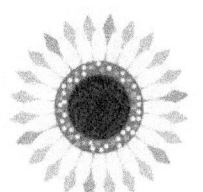

---

1 courgette

1 tbsp tomato puree

1 veg stock cube

Splash of red wine

Italian herbs

3 cups of pasta shapes

Fresh basil

10 sticks of Asparagus

5-6 chestnut mushrooms

Method:

1. chop all veg including tomatoes and garlic and place on a baking tray with olive oil and place in the oven to bake for approx. 15-20mins

2. when veg is baked add it all to a pan, and add tin of tomatoes, tomato puree, veg stock and Italian herbs

3. Boil some pasta shapes.

4. Add a splash of red wine to the sauce, and stir.

5. Lightly fry asparagus and mushroom's in a separate pan.

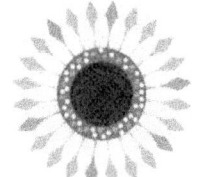

1/2 cup raspberries

1 tablespoon maca, goji berries, aloe & hemp

Method:

Blend it all and serve.

Source references:

** Preliminary evidence that vegetarian diet improves mood. American Public Health Association annual conference, November 7-11, 2009. Philadelphia, PA.

** Effect of a single high-fat meal on endothelial function in healthy subjects. Am J Cardiol. 1997 Feb 1; 79(3):350-4.

** The capacity of foodstuffs to induce innate immune activation of human monocytes in vitro is dependent on food content of stimulants of Toll-like receptors 2 and 4. Br J Nutr. 2011 Jan; 105(1):15-23.

** The capacity of foodstuffs to induce innate immune activation of human monocytes in vitro is dependent on food content of stimulants of Toll-like receptors 2 and 4. Br J Nutr. 2011 Jan; 105(1):15-23.

** Dietary fatty acids and pancreatic cancer in the NIH-AARP diet and health study. J Natl Cancer Inst. 2009 Jul 15;101(14):1001-11.

** Egg consumption and the risk of cancer: a multisite case-control study in Uruguay.

** Nitrites, nitrosamines, and cancer. Lancet. 1968 May 18;1(7551):1071-2.

** Multidrug-Resistant Staphylococcus aureus in US Meat and Poultry. Clin Infect Dis. 2011 May;52(10):1227-30.

** Knutsen SF. Lifestyle and the use of health services. Am J Clin Nutr. 1994 May;59(5 Suppl):1171S-1175S.

** Canadian Cancer Registries Epidemiology Research Group. Salt, processed meat and the risk of cancer. Eur J Cancer Prev. 2011 Mar;20(2):132-9.

** Consumption of meat and dairy and lymphoma risk in the European Prospective Investigation into Cancer and Nutrition. Int J Cancer. 2011 Feb 1;128(3):623-34.

** Detection of exogenous and endogenous avian leukosis virus in commercial chicken eggs using reverse transcription and polymerase chain reaction assay. Avian Pathology (1999) 28, 385±392

** Consumption of cured meats and prospective risk of chronic obstructive pulmonary disease in women. Am J Clin Nutr. 2008 Apr;87(4):1002-8.

** Animal protein intake and risk of inflammatory bowel disease: The E3N prospective study. Am J Gastroenterol. 2010 Oct; 105(10):2195-201.

** Associations of diet with albuminuria and kidney function decline. Clin J Am Soc Nephrol. 2010 May; 5(5):836-43.

** Food groups and risk of benign prostatic hyperplasia. Urology. 2006 Jan;67(1):73-9.

** Plasma and erythrocyte biomarkers of dairy fat intake and risk of ischemic heart disease. American Journal of Clinical Nutrition, 86(4):929, 2007.

** Animal food intake and cooking methods in relation to endometrial cancer risk in shanghai. Br. J. Cancer, 95(11):15861592, 2006.

** Diet-induced metabolic acidosis. Clin Nutr 2011 30(4):416 – 421.

** Sympathetic nervous system activity and resting metabolic rate in vegetarians. Metab. Clin. Exp. 1994 43(5):621 – 625.

** Long-term low-calorie low-protein vegan diet and endurance exercise are associated with low cardiometabolic risk. Rejuvenation Res. 2007 10(2):225 – 234.

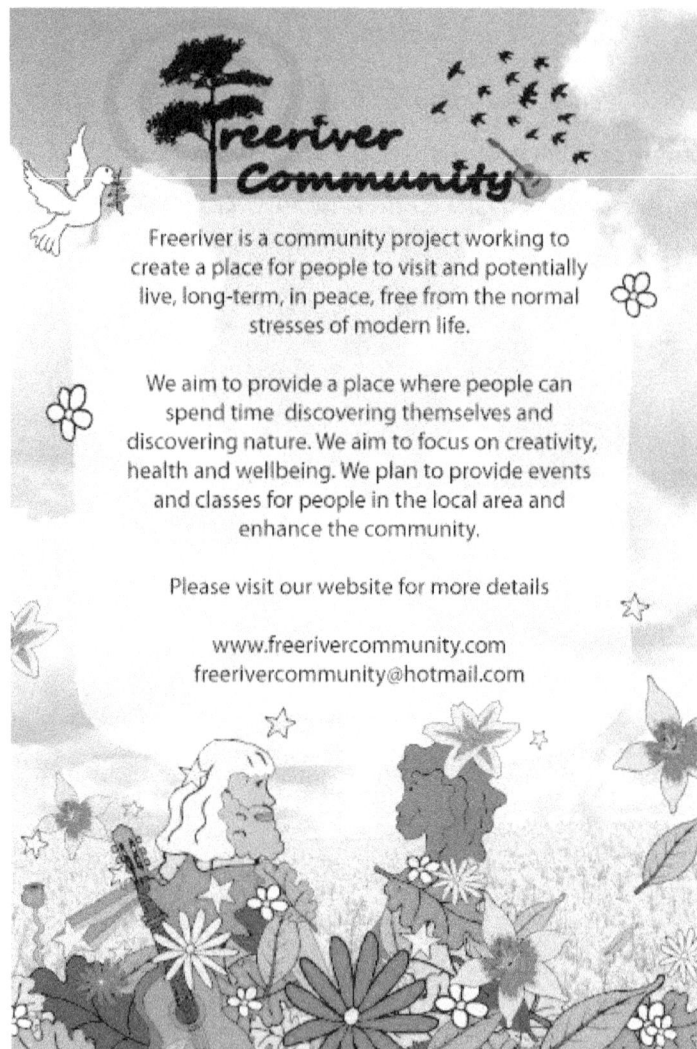

Freeriver is a community project working to create a place for people to visit and potentially live, long-term, in peace, free from the normal stresses of modern life.

We aim to provide a place where people can spend time discovering themselves and discovering nature. We aim to focus on creativity, health and wellbeing. We plan to provide events and classes for people in the local area and enhance the community.

Please visit our website for more details

www.freerivercommunity.com
freerivercommunity@hotmail.com

Freeriver is a project that is currently underway to create a place for people to visit

and maybe to live in peace, free from the normal stresses of modern life.

Its aim is to provide a place where people can spend time discovering themselves

and discovering nature, focus on creativity, health and well-being. to provide events

and classes for people in the local area and enhance the community.

Please visit the website for more details

WWW.FREERIVERCOMMUNITY.COM

FREERIVERCOMMUNITY@HOTMAIL.COM